STRONG IN 30

Resistance Training for Weight Loss

30-Minute Workouts to Burn Fat, Build

Muscle, and Transform Your Body

STRONG IN 30

Resistance Training for Weight Loss
30-Minute Workouts to Burn Fat, Build
Muscle, and Transform Your Body

Ryan Cole

Trade Paperback ISBN: 978-1-954921-07-8
eISBN: 978-1-954921-06-1
Library of Congress Control Number: available upon request

Summit Publishing
Chicago, IL

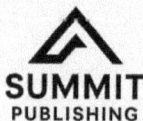

SUMMIT
PUBLISHING

Dedication

To everyone whoever thought they were too busy to change — you'll find the time, and it will change your life

Table of Contents

Introduction – Why 30 Minutes Is Enough

My Story: From Frustration to Breakthrough

I didn't always have fitness figured out. In fact, for years, I was stuck in the same cycle most people know all too well: endless cardio sessions, strict diets that felt impossible to maintain, and quick-fix gadgets that promised results but left me disappointed. I remember grinding away on treadmills and bikes, drenched in sweat, only to step on the scale and see almost no change. The frustration was crushing. At times, I wondered if maybe my body just wasn't built to lose weight.

The turning point came when I picked up a set of dumbbells. For the first time, I wasn't just out of breath—I felt my muscles working. A few weeks later, my clothes fit differently, even though the scale barely moved. That's when I realized the truth: the number on the scale isn't the full story. Resistance training wasn't just helping me burn calories—it was reshaping my body, boosting my metabolism, and building a confidence I hadn't felt in years.

Why Resistance Training + 30 Minutes Works

Here's the best part: this transformation didn't require hours in the gym. It required smart, focused sessions—just 30 minutes, a few times per week.

Science confirms what I discovered through experience:

- **Efficiency beats duration** – Short, intense resistance sessions stimulate muscle growth and calorie burn long after the workout ends.

- **Consistency is sustainable** – 30 minutes fits into even the busiest schedules, making it far easier to stick with.

- **Recovery is built in** – Unlike punishing 2-hour sessions, shorter workouts give your body the time it needs to repair and grow stronger.

In other words: it's not about doing more—it's about doing what works.

Why Most People Struggle (and How This Fixes It)

If you've ever felt frustrated by weight loss, it's probably because you:

- Relied too much on cardio, only to plateau.
- Tried fad diets that left you drained and hungry.
- Believed you needed endless time at the gym to see results.

This book is about breaking that cycle. Instead of extreme

routines or gimmicks, it gives you a clear, proven system: resistance training + smart nutrition + consistency. Together, they create natural, sustainable fat loss and lasting strength.

What You'll Learn in This Book

By the time you finish, you'll understand:

1. **The science of resistance training** and why it beats cardio for weight loss.

2. **How sets, reps, and recovery work**—the real building blocks of strength and fat loss.

3. **Why muscle burns fat even at rest**, and how to harness this effect.

4. **Nutrition basics that fuel results** without restrictive dieting.

5. **Multiple 30-minute workout blueprints**—for dumbbells, bands, and bodyweight—so you're covered anywhere.

6. **How to stay motivated and consistent**, even on days when you don't feel like showing up.

A Lifestyle, Not a Phase

This book isn't about a "6-week shred" or punishing yourself into shape. It's about building a lifestyle where:

- You wake up with more energy.

- You feel strong and capable in your body.

- You enjoy the process instead of dreading it.

Think of this as your roadmap to lasting change. It's not about chasing perfection—it's about progress, one 30-minute session at a time.

WHY 30 MINUTES WORKS

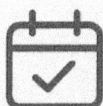

EFFICIENCY
Short sessions build muscle and burn calories

CONSISTENCY
30 minutes is easier to fit into a busy day

RECOVERY
Less time exercising allows better repair

Coach's Note

I've been where you are: frustrated, tired, and unsure where to start. But I promise you this—you don't need to overhaul your entire life to get results. You just need the right system, and the belief that progress compounds. Every rep, every set, every walk adds up.

My hope is that as you read, you'll begin to see yourself differently. Not as someone "trying to lose weight," but as someone building strength, health, and confidence—one workout at a time.

Inspirational Quote

"Don't limit your challenges. Challenge your limits." – Unknown

Chapter 1 – What Is Resistance Training?

When most people hear the word *workout*, they picture endless jogging on a treadmill or sweating through a spin class. That's what I thought too when I was first trying to lose weight. I believed the only way to get results was to do more cardio, burn more calories, and keep pushing until the fat melted away.

But here's the truth I wish I had known earlier: **resistance training is the real secret weapon.** It doesn't just burn calories during a workout—it reshapes your body, builds strength, and turns you into a more efficient fat-burning machine long after you've left the gym.

A Short History of Resistance Training

Resistance training isn't new. Ancient civilizations used it to prepare for war and survival.

- Greek athletes lifted stones to build strength for competitions.

- Roman soldiers trained with heavier weapons than

they actually used in battle so they'd be faster and stronger in real combat.

- Ancient Indian wrestlers swung heavy clubs to build functional strength and resilience.

The principle hasn't changed in thousands of years: when you challenge your muscles with resistance, they adapt and grow stronger. Today, resistance training has moved from ancient battlefields to gyms, homes, and parks—but the benefits are still universal. It's the closest thing we have to a time-tested formula for getting stronger, leaner, and healthier.

What Resistance Training Really Means

Resistance training simply means exercising your muscles against some kind of force. That force could be:

- Free weights (dumbbells, barbells, kettlebells)

- Resistance bands

- Your own body weight (push-ups, squats, planks)

- Machines at the gym

The goal is the same: to challenge your muscles so they adapt, grow stronger, and burn more calories—even when you're not working out.

Think about it like this: when you lift a dumbbell, you're telling your body, *"Hey, I need more strength for this task."*

Your body responds by repairing your muscles and making them stronger for next time.

🎁 Sidebar: Science Spotlight

- A 2019 study in *Mayo Clinic Proceedings* found that **strength training reduced the risk of death from all causes by 23%**, independent of cardio.

- Resistance training is linked to **better insulin sensitivity**, meaning your body uses food for fuel instead of storing it as fat.

- Even two short lifting sessions per week have been shown to reduce age-related muscle loss.

☞ Bottom line: lifting doesn't just help you look better—it helps you *live better and longer*.

The Science Behind Resistance Training

Here's why it's powerful:

1. **Progressive Overload** – When you gradually increase the resistance (more weight, more reps, or slower tempo), your muscles adapt and grow.

2. **Muscle = Metabolism** – Muscle tissue is "active tissue." A pound of muscle burns more calories at rest than a pound of fat. This means you're not just getting stronger—you're boosting your body's

ability to burn fat 24/7.

3. **Longevity Factor** – Studies show resistance training helps prevent age-related muscle loss, improves bone density, and reduces risk of injuries.

4. **Hormonal Benefits** – Lifting stimulates growth hormone and testosterone, both of which help with fat burning and muscle building. It also improves insulin sensitivity, which makes it easier for your body to use food for energy instead of storing it as fat.

5. **Brain & Mood Boost** – Research shows resistance training reduces stress, sharpens focus, and can help fight anxiety and depression.

In other words, resistance training isn't just about looking good—it's about building a body and mind that work for you for decades to come.

But Don't I Need Cardio Too?

You might be wondering: *"What about cardio?"*

Here's the thing: cardio is good for your heart and lungs, but it doesn't reshape your body the way resistance training does. Cardio burns calories during the activity. Resistance training builds muscle that keeps burning calories after the activity—for hours, sometimes days.

And here's a personal note: I prefer walking instead of running or long cardio sessions. Walking is lower impact, less stressful on your joints, and actually lowers your stress hormone levels. Science backs this up—walking regularly has been shown to improve fat loss and overall health more consistently than high-intensity cardio for many people. Running can increase appetite and fatigue, while walking keeps you consistent and motivated.

The "Bulky" Myth

A lot of people, especially women, hesitate to start resistance training because they fear they'll get "too bulky." Let's clear that up right now:

- Women generally don't have enough testosterone to build large, bulky muscles like male bodybuilders. What lifting does is **tone and shape the body— making you look leaner, not bigger.**

- Men who want to look like professional bodybuilders have to spend years training intensely, eating enormous amounts of food, and sometimes using performance enhancers. Simply lifting weights 2–4 times a week will not suddenly make you oversized.

- What lifting *will* do is make your body firmer, your posture better, and your metabolism stronger.

So if you're worried about "bulking up," don't be. Resistance training builds the kind of muscle that makes you look lean, athletic, and confident.

Practical Starter Advice

If you're new, here's how to start:

- **Frequency:** Begin with 2 days a week. Once that feels good, move to 3–4 days.
- **Equipment:** You don't need a gym. Start with your bodyweight. Add dumbbells or bands when you're ready.
- **Form first:** Always focus on proper form before adding weight. Good form prevents injury and makes the exercise more effective.
- **Progress slowly:** Add small amounts of weight or extra reps over time. Consistency matters more than speed.

Even short sessions work. **Twenty minutes of resistance training + a short walk can deliver amazing results** if you stick with it.

🎁 Sidebar: Beginner FAQs

Q: What if I've never lifted before?
A: Start with bodyweight moves (squats, push-ups, planks). They teach control and build a foundation.

Q: Am I too old to start?
A: Absolutely not. Resistance training is one of the best ways to preserve independence and strength as you age. Studies show people in their 70s and 80s still gain muscle when lifting.

Q: Do I need supplements?

A: No. Whole foods and consistency matter more. Supplements are optional.

Coach's Note

When I started, I was scared of the weight room. I thought lifting weights would make me bulky, or that I didn't "belong" there. But once I picked up that first dumbbell and stuck with it, my body and confidence changed.

I remember my first month: the scale barely moved, but I noticed my jeans fitting looser and my arms looking firmer. That was when I realized resistance training was different from everything else I had tried. It wasn't about chasing a number—it was about changing how my body looked and felt.

You don't need to lift heavy right away. Start light, focus on good form, and build from there. Remember: even 2 days a week of resistance training is enough to see results when you're starting out. Once you're comfortable, aim for 3–4 days. And if you miss a day, don't beat yourself up. Just pick it back up the next day. What matters most is staying consistent over time.

Inspirational Quote

"Strength does not come from winning. Your struggles develop your strengths. When you go through hardships and decide not to surrender, that is strength." – Arnold Schwarzenegger

Chapter 2 – Why Resistance Training Beats Cardio for Weight Loss

If you've ever tried to lose weight, you've probably heard this advice: *"Just do more cardio."* For years, I believed it too. I ran, biked, swam—you name it. And while I did lose some weight, the results never lasted. As soon as I slowed down the cardio, the weight crept right back.

That's because cardio is only part of the puzzle. If your goal is to burn fat, lose weight naturally, and keep it off, **resistance training beats cardio every single time.**

Cardio: The Short-Term Burner

When you jog, bike, or take a spin class, you burn calories. For example:

- Jogging for 30 minutes burns ~250–300 calories.

- Cycling for 30 minutes burns ~200–400 calories (depending on intensity).

That's not bad, but here's the catch: **when the workout ends, the burn mostly stops.** Your body goes back to its normal rate. You only burned during the activity itself.

Even worse? Your body adapts to cardio. The more you do, the more efficient your body becomes—meaning you burn fewer calories for the same workout. This is why so many people hit a plateau: at first the pounds come off, but eventually progress stalls unless you go longer and harder. Too much cardio can even backfire by breaking down muscle tissue—which slows your metabolism.

Resistance Training: The Long-Term Fat Burner

Now compare that to resistance training. A 30-minute lifting workout might not burn as many calories during the session as a run—but the magic happens after.

Here's why resistance training is the game-changer:

1. **Afterburn Effect (EPOC):** When you lift weights, your body uses extra oxygen to repair your muscles. This recovery burns calories for 24–48 hours—even while you're at work, watching TV, or sleeping.

2. **Muscle Growth = Faster Metabolism:** Every pound of muscle burns calories at rest, all day, every day. Think of muscle as a built-in furnace—the more you have, the hotter your metabolism runs.

3. **Body Recomposition:** Cardio alone might make you smaller, but resistance training reshapes you. You lose fat and gain lean muscle, creating that athletic,

toned look.

4. **Hormonal Boost:** Lifting improves insulin
   sensitivity (helping your body use carbs as fuel
   instead of storing them as fat), raises growth
   hormone, and balances stress hormones.

☞ In short: cardio burns calories while you do it.
Resistance training teaches your body to burn calories
around the clock.

CARDIO vs. RESISTANCE TRAINING
THE CLEAR DIFFERENCE

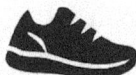

CALORIES BURNED

✓ **Cardio:** Burns more calories during the workout (e.g, running 30 min = 300 calories).

✗ **Afterburn Effect (EPOC)** Minimal afterburn, calorie burn stops when workout ends.

✗ **Muscle & Metabolism** Builds endurance but can break down muscle if overdone, slowing metabolism.

✗ **Body Composition** May make you smaller but often leads to 'skinny-fat' (less muscle, higher fat %).

✗ **Hormonal Effects** Can increase corfisol (stress hormone) if excessive, leading to more cravings and belly fat.

✗ **Sustainability** Effective shori-term but can lead to plateaus and burnout.

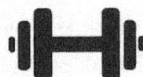

RESISTANCE TRAINING

✓ Triggers muscle repair and recovery, burning extra calories well affer the session.

✓ Builds lean muscle, which raises resting metabolism- helping you burn fat 24/7.

✓ Reshapess the body- toned, firm, and athietic.

Boosts growth hormone & testosterone (in both men and women). improving fat loss, muscle gain, and mood.

✓ Sustainable long-term; fewer workouts still deliver results due to muscle- building effects.

Bottom Line:

Cardio = Calorie burning now

Resistance Training = Calorie burning now + later, with muscie-building benefits that last

Do both–but make resistance training your foundation.

🎁 Sidebar: Why Cardio Can Backfire

- Too much cardio + calorie restriction = muscle loss.
- Less muscle = slower metabolism.
- Slower metabolism = easier fat gain later.

This is why many people yo-yo with weight loss: cardio + diet makes them smaller for a short time, but once they stop, the weight rebounds—often worse than before.

The Appetite Connection

Cardio often spikes hunger. If you've ever finished a long run and then wanted to eat everything in sight, you know the feeling. Many people end up eating back the calories they just burned.

Resistance training works differently. Because it emphasizes muscle growth and pairs so well with higher-protein eating, it helps keep hunger more stable. You feel fuller, stronger, and less likely to binge. That makes sticking to a calorie deficit much easier.

Walking vs. Running: The Smarter "In-Between"

Now, don't get me wrong—I'm not anti-cardio. But I've learned something important: **walking is better than running for most people starting out.**

Why walking wins:

- **Low impact:** Doesn't pound your joints.

- **Steadier appetite:** Running often spikes hunger; walking usually doesn't.

- **Stress reducing:** Walking lowers cortisol (the belly-fat hormone).

- **Sustainable:** You're more likely to walk daily than commit to running long distances.

That's why I recommend walking on your non-lifting days. It complements resistance training perfectly, helps recovery, and burns fat without the crash.

The Psychological Edge of Lifting

Here's something people don't talk about enough: lifting gives you visible proof of progress. With cardio, it's harder to see change beyond stamina. With resistance training, you notice muscles firming, strength improving, clothes fitting differently.

That feedback loop builds confidence—and confidence fuels consistency. It's a cycle that makes resistance training easier to stick with long-term.

Coach's Note

When I switched from endless cardio to resistance training, everything changed. My energy went up, I slept better, and I broke free from the cycle of "lose weight, gain it back."

I also noticed something surprising: after cardio, I was starving. I'd undo half my work by overeating. After lifting, especially with enough protein, I felt satisfied—not ravenous. That alone made it easier to stay on track.

And don't underestimate walking. Adding daily walks— especially outdoors—gave me recovery, stress relief, and calorie burn without exhaustion. Between lifting and walking, I finally found a rhythm I could stick with for life.

Inspirational Quote

"Suffer the pain of discipline or suffer the pain of regret." – Unknown

Chapter 3 – Sets, Reps, Rest, and Recovery Explained

When I first started lifting, I was lost when people threw around terms like "3 sets of 12" or "progressive overload." I remember standing in the gym with a plan in my hand thinking: *"What does this even mean?"*

The good news is this: once you understand sets, reps, and rest, the whole world of resistance training starts to make sense. These are the building blocks of every effective workout. Master them, and you'll never feel lost in the gym again.

What Are Reps?

A **rep** (short for repetition) is one complete movement of an exercise.

Examples:

- One push-up = one rep

- One squat = one rep

- One bicep curl up and down = one rep

The **rep range** you choose determines the result:

- **1–6 reps** → **Strength** (heavy weights, longer rest)

- **8–12 reps** → **Muscle Growth (Hypertrophy)**

- **12–20 reps** → **Endurance** (lighter weight, higher reps, shorter rest)

☞ Think of reps as the "language" of resistance training. Once you understand them, every program makes sense.

What Are Sets?

A **set** is a group of reps performed in sequence before resting.

Example:

- Do 10 push-ups in a row → that's **1 set of 10**.

- Rest, then do 10 more → that's **2 sets of 10**.

Most beginner workouts use **2–4 sets per exercise**, which is enough to challenge the body and build progress.

How Long Should You Rest Between Sets?

Rest isn't wasted time—it's when your muscles reload. How much you rest depends on your goal:

- **Strength (1–6 reps):** 2–5 minutes (heavier weights need longer recovery)

- **Muscle Growth (8–12 reps):** 60–90 seconds (enough to recover, but still keep muscles under tension)

- **Endurance (12–20 reps):** 30–60 seconds (short rest keeps heart rate high)

☞ **Pro Tip:** Beginners often rush through sets thinking shorter rest = better workout. In reality, resting the right amount makes your next set stronger and more effective.

The Science of What's Happening Inside

Each style of training stresses your body differently:

- **Strength Training (1–6 reps):** Heavy lifting recruits fast-twitch fibers and challenges the nervous system. You get stronger without necessarily looking bigger.

- **Hypertrophy (8–12 reps):** Creates microtears in muscle fibers. During recovery, the body repairs them with protein, making them larger and denser.

- **Endurance (12–20 reps):** Improves how your muscles use oxygen, boosting stamina and fatigue resistance.

Think of it like this:

- Strength = teaching your muscles to fire harder.

- Hypertrophy = making your muscles bigger.

- Endurance = teaching your muscles to last longer.

REP RANGES AND GOALS

STRENGTH	HYPERTROPHY	ENDURANCE
1–6 REPS	8–12 REPS	12–20 REPS
HEAVY	MODERATE	LIGHT
LONG REST	60–90s REST	30–60s REST

Progressive Overload: The Secret Ingredient

If sets and reps are the building blocks, **progressive overload** is the blueprint. It means gradually challenging your muscles more over time.

Ways to apply overload:

- Add a small amount of weight.

- Increase reps at the same weight.
- Add an extra set.
- Slow down tempo (3–4 seconds lowering phase).
- Shorten rest periods slightly.

Without overload, your body adapts and plateaus. With it, you keep growing stronger, leaner, and more capable.

🎁 Sidebar: Common Beginner Mistakes

1. **Not resting enough** → leads to weaker sets.

2. **Going too heavy too soon** → poor form + higher risk of injury.

3. **Random rep ranges** → stick with ranges that match your goals.

4. **Overtraining** → remember, growth happens during recovery, not the workout.

Chapter 3 Sets, Reps, Rest, and Recovery

One day at the gym, I looked at my workout sheet and saw "3x12" written next to an exercise. I had no idea what that meant, (Was hat a typo?) If you're also confused by all this lifting lingo, don't worry. Let's clear it up.

Reps = Repetitions of an exercise, (Lifting the weight and lowering it counts as one rep.)

Sets = A group of repetitions repeated a certain number of times. (E.g, 3 sets of 12 reps each,)

Rest = The amount of time to rest between sets. (The shorter the rest, the more challenging the workout.)

Goal	Reps	Rest	Rest
Strength	1–6	2–5 min.	2–5 sec.
Hypertrophy	8–12	60–90 secs.	60–90 secos.
Endurance	15+	30–60 secs.	30–60 secos.

Progressive overload is the master key to success in the gym.

Add reps → Add~~onceative~~ → Add tempo → Add sets

Recovery matters.

COACH'S NOTE:
In my early days. I didn't progress because I never gave my body time to recover. Rest. nutrition, and sleep are non-negotiable for gains.

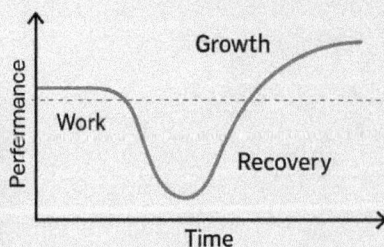

"Consistency is the key to success."

–John Wooden

3

Why Rest and Recovery Matter

Here's the truth: when you lift weights, you're not "building" muscle—you're breaking it down. Growth happens **after** the workout, during rest and recovery.

Types of rest:

- **Between sets:** See guidelines above.

- **Between workouts:** Give each muscle group at least one day off before training it again. Most people progress best on 3–4 training days per week, not 7.

☞ Even 2 days a week is enough to start seeing results.

Recovery: The Hidden Workout

Recovery is as important as training. It includes:

- **Sleep:** At least 7–8 hours. During deep sleep, your body releases growth hormone, repairs muscle, and burns fat.

- **Nutrition:** Protein is your repair material (more in Chapter 5).

- **Active Recovery:** Walk on off days. It promotes circulation, reduces soreness, and keeps you moving.

Think of recovery like charging your phone: if you never plug it in, it dies. Ignore recovery, and your body will burn out the same way.

Coach's Note

When I finally understood sets, reps, and rest, my training changed completely. I went from random, frustrating workouts to structured sessions that delivered results.

I used to believe "more was better"—more sets, heavier weight, less rest. But that only left me exhausted and stuck. Once I respected rest and followed progressive overload, everything improved: strength, energy, and body composition.

Personally, I've found **8–12 reps per set with 60–90 seconds rest** is the sweet spot for fat loss and muscle tone. It's intense enough to build lean muscle but short enough to keep my heart rate up.

If your goal is to tone up, start here. Be patient, be consistent, and remember: recovery isn't weakness—it's the fuel for your next breakthrough.

Inspirational Quote

"Consistency is the key to success" – John Wooden

Chapter 4 – Why Resistance Training Keeps Burning Calories After the Workout Is Over

I'll never forget the first time I learned about something called the **afterburn effect**. I was blown away. The idea that I could finish a workout, take a shower, eat dinner, and still be burning calories afterward? That felt like discovering a cheat code for fat loss.

Here's the truth: resistance training is one of the most powerful ways to make that happen.

The Afterburn Effect (EPOC) Explained

The scientific name is **Excess Post-Exercise Oxygen Consumption (EPOC)**.

When you finish a challenging workout, your body doesn't just shut down and relax. Instead, it has a recovery checklist to work through:

- Rebuild and repair muscle fibers

- Replenish energy stores (glycogen)

- Restore oxygen levels in blood and tissues

- Clear out metabolic waste (like lactate)

- Rebalance hormones (stress, growth, recovery)

All of this takes energy—meaning your metabolism stays elevated for hours after the workout.

💡 Studies show metabolism can stay elevated for **24–48 hours** after strength training. That's like getting bonus calorie burn while you sleep, work, or watch TV.

Think of it like this:

- **Cardio = paying cash** (calories burned during the workout).

- **Resistance training = using a credit card** (calories burned during and after, as your body "pays down" the recovery debt).

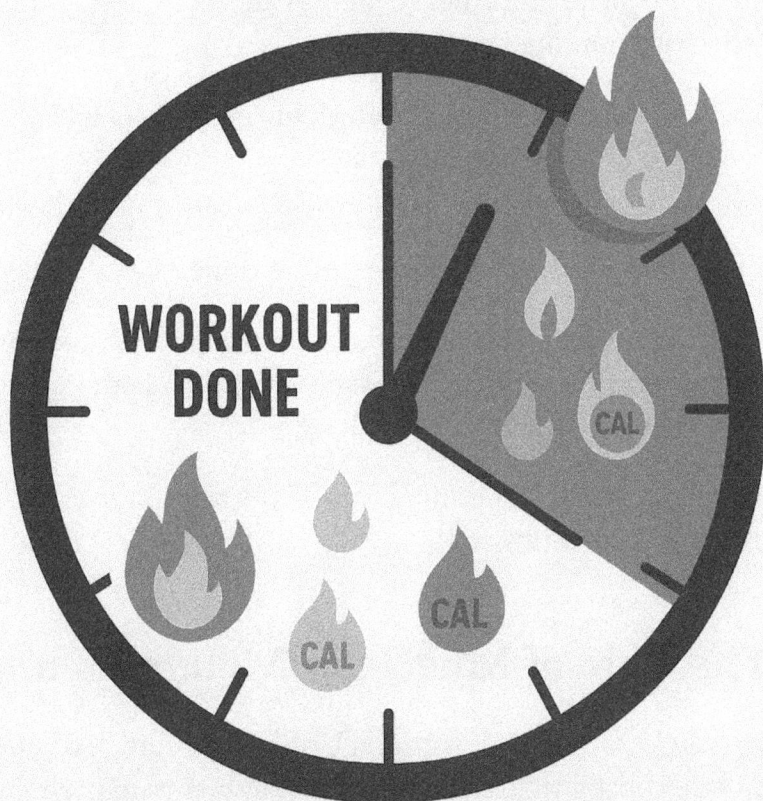

STILL BURNING CALORIES HOURS LATER

WORKOUT DONE

24-48 HOURS

Why Resistance Training Beats Steady-State Cardio

Don't get me wrong—cardio is great for your heart and lungs. But when it comes to fat loss and body reshaping, resistance training has the edge.

- **Cardio (running, cycling):** Burns calories while you're moving, then stops.

- **Resistance training:** Burns calories while you're moving, and long after you're done.

Plus, cardio doesn't build muscle the way lifting does. And remember: muscle is active tissue that keeps your metabolism humming all day long.

☞ In short: cardio is renting calorie burn; resistance training is investing in it.

The Role of Muscle in Metabolism

Muscle is your body's furnace. Unlike fat (storage tissue), muscle constantly burns energy just to maintain itself.

Here's a simple comparison:
- 1 pound of fat burns about **2 calories/day at rest**
- 1 pound of muscle burns about **6–10 calories/day at rest**

That might sound small, but it adds up. If you gain 5 pounds of lean muscle, you'll burn an extra **50 calories a day** just sitting still. Over a year, that's about **18,000**

calories, or roughly **5 pounds of fat lost**—without doing anything extra.

☞ Building and maintaining muscle isn't just about looking fit. It's the most natural way to speed up your metabolism.

Sleep and Recovery: Your Hidden Fat-Burning Allies

Here's something most people miss: the magic of resistance training doesn't just happen in the gym—it happens while you rest.

During deep sleep, your body:

- Releases **growth hormone**, essential for muscle repair and fat burning

- Repairs micro-tears in muscle fibers, making them stronger

- Balances hunger hormones (ghrelin & leptin), reducing cravings

- Lowers cortisol (stress hormone linked to belly fat)

Skipping sleep is like throwing away half the benefits of your workout. If you want to maximize fat loss, make **7–8 hours of quality sleep** part of your plan.

Walking Between Workouts

Here's the surprising part: you don't need to crush yourself with cardio on "off" days. Walking is the perfect complement to resistance training.

Why?

- Low impact → gentle on joints

- Recovery booster → improves blood flow to sore muscles

- Stress reducer → lowers cortisol, which helps burn fat

- Fat-focused → at low intensity, the body uses fat as its primary fuel

☞ I call walking the "silent multiplier." It makes your training results bigger without draining your energy.

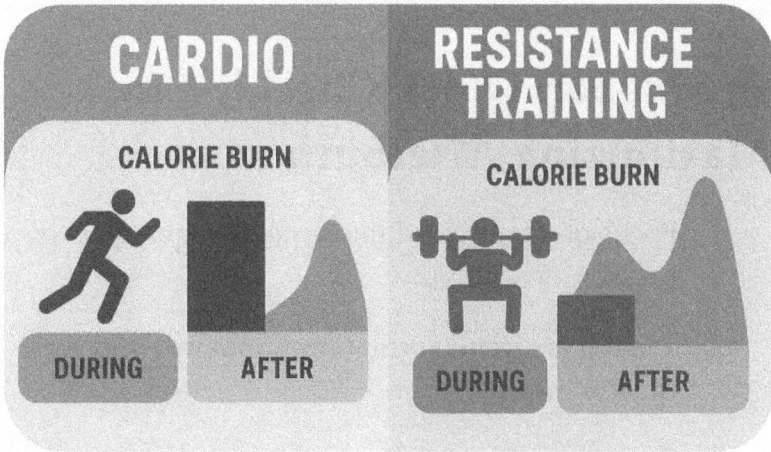

Practical Example: Cardio vs. Resistance Training

Let's compare two 30-minute workouts:

30-Minute Run

- Burns ~300 calories

- Burn stops when you stop

30-Minute Resistance Workout

- Burns ~250 calories during the workout

- Burns another ~150 calories in recovery (EPOC)

- Builds muscle → burns more calories at rest every day

Result? Resistance training wins for both short-term and long-term fat loss.

🎁 Sidebar: Quick Checklist for Maximizing Afterburn

1. Focus on **compound movements** (squats, rows, presses, deadlifts).

2. Train in a **circuit format** (minimal rest, multiple muscle groups).

3. Push intensity—challenge yourself, but keep good form.

4. Prioritize recovery (protein, hydration, sleep).

5. Add **daily walking** to keep metabolism elevated on off days.

Coach's Note

When I only did cardio, I was always stuck in the same cycle: progress for a few weeks, then plateau. If I missed a run, my calorie burn stopped—and so did my fat loss.

When I switched to resistance training, the game changed. My body kept burning calories even after the workout. I started looking leaner, feeling stronger, and staying more consistent—because I could see results faster and with less burnout.

☞ My advice: don't chase hours of cardio. Start with **2–3 resistance workouts a week**, walk daily, and focus on recovery. That's the real fat-loss formula.

Inspirational Quote

"Strength does not come from the body. It comes from the will." – Arnold Schwarzenegger

Chapter 5 – Nutrition for Fat Loss and Muscle Growth

If your workouts are the **engine of transformation**, your nutrition is the **fuel**. You can train as hard as you want, but if your eating habits don't support your goals, you'll always feel like you're pushing a car uphill with the brakes on.

I know this firsthand. Early in my journey, I tried every fad diet out there: low-carb, keto, juice cleanses, meal-replacement shakes, even skipping meals altogether. Sometimes I dropped a few pounds, but it never lasted. What finally worked wasn't extreme—it was understanding how calories, protein, carbs, fats, and habits actually influence weight loss and muscle growth.

CHAPTER 5

NUTRITION FOR FAT LOSS AND MUSCLE GROWTH

If workouts are the engine of transformation, nutrition is the fuel. You can't out train a poor diet. No matter how consistent your workours are, if your eating habdian't align with your goals, progress is vill feel slow, frustrating and unsustainable. This chapter is about giving you the sáme fotion–simple, proven nuurcition.

Calories In vs. Calories Out (CICO)

At its core, weight management comes down to energy balance:

- Calories In = food and drink you consume + workouts, daily activities + body function (*breathing. digestion*)

- A consistent calorie 500 calories defcst of about 500 calories per week.

But here's ane nualise muca as principles to nutrition,

Protein: The Muscle Builder

Prioritize protein–prüorritlze protein:

- Provides the building ттг:
  = 0 7–10 grams per pound of body weight per day)–=

- Gats you µtall ongeremansully = 30g̃

Axmpεct al is mֈcn añ as quucd' as:

Protein: The Muscle Builder

Carbs and Eats: Energy and Hormone Helpers

- Complex carbs (oals, rice, beans, potatoes, truit) → slow-degesting, steady energy; fast energy but easy to overeat

- Hydrotation can help hormones &

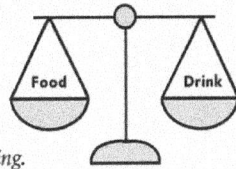

50 calories of candy, fish, or poultry = *25–30 g

Protein portion side (a plim-sized porrion of meat, fish, or poultrv) = *20–30g

I scoop **protein** power = 20–26g

> Keep fats thotldenrtrests

Mindset: Fuel vs. Treats

Pizza, burgers, sweets =, purgese, Lean proteins, whole carbs, colorful vegetables – fuel.

A target: 30–90ŕ̇ nuir tious meals, 10–20% treats:

* *Take care* of your body. It's the only place you have to live.

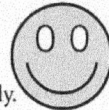

Calories In vs. Calories Out (CICO)

At the foundation of weight management is energy balance:

- **Calories in** = food and drink you consume

- **Calories out** = energy you burn through workouts, daily activity, and basic survival functions (breathing, digestion, brain function)

If you eat **more** than you burn → you gain weight.
If you eat **less** than you burn → you lose weight.

☞ To lose about 1 pound of fat per week, you need a deficit of ~3,500 calories, or about 500 per day.

But here's the nuance: not all calories feel the same.

- **500 calories of fast food** → digests quickly, spikes hunger, leaves you tired.

- **500 calories of whole foods** (chicken, rice, veggies) → fills you up, fuels workouts, supports recovery.

The goal isn't starvation—it's creating a manageable deficit while still fueling strength and energy.

The Power of Protein

If there's one nutrient that deserves your focus, it's **protein**.

Why protein is king:

- Repairs and rebuilds muscles after workouts

- Keeps you full and satisfied (easier to stay in a deficit)

- Burns more calories during digestion (highest thermic effect of food)

💡 **Aim for 0.7–1.0 grams of protein per pound of bodyweight per day.**
Example: If you weigh 180 lbs → target 125–180g protein daily.

Protein Sources

- **Animal-based:** Chicken, turkey, lean beef, fish, eggs, Greek yogurt

- **Plant-based:** Beans, lentils, tofu, tempeh, seitan

- **Convenient:** Protein shakes or bars (useful, but not required)

Protein Myths (Busted)

- *"Too much protein harms kidneys."* → No evidence in healthy people.

- *"You can't absorb more than 30g at once."* → False; your body uses it over time.

☞ Pro Tip: Spread protein across meals instead of saving it all for dinner. Muscles need steady fuel all day.

Carbs and Fats: The Co-Stars

While protein is the star, carbs and fats are essential co-stars.

Carbohydrates

- Your main fuel source during workouts.

- **Complex carbs:** Oats, brown rice, potatoes, fruit = steady energy.

- **Simple carbs:** Sweets, soda, pastries = quick spikes, easy to overeat.
  ☞ Best rule: eat mostly complex carbs, save simple carbs for quick pre- or post-workout boosts.

Fats

- Vital for hormones, brain function, and recovery.

- **Healthy fats:** Avocado, nuts, olive oil, fatty fish.

- **Avoid:** Trans fats (processed fried foods, packaged snacks).
  ☞ Keep fats moderate: too little wrecks hormones; too much crowds out protein.

💧 HYDRATION

Water is the most underrated performance booster. Even mild dehydration (as little as 2% of bodyweight) can hurt strength, endurance, and focus.

Daily target: About half your body weight (lbs) in ounces of water.

Example: 180 lbs = -90 oz. water/day

Pro tip: Spread it throughout the day, not all at once. Add electrolytes on hot days or during sweaty workouts.

Coach's Tip: Supplements can fill small gaps, but they can't replace a balanced diet, quality sleep, and consistent training. Think of them as the finishing touches on the foundation you've already built.

🏅 SUPPLEMENTS

💊 ESSENTIAL

Protein Powder (Whey, Casein, Plant-Based)
Convenient way to reach daily protein goals, especially post-workout.

Electrolytes (Sodium, Potassium, Magnesium)
Helpful if you sweat heavily or train in hot climates.

Caffeine (Coffee or Pre-Workout)
Boosts focus and endurance, but not essential. Use sparingly to avoid dependency.

BCAAs / EAAs
(Branched/Essential Amino Acids)
Useful mainly if you train fasted or struggle to hit protein goals.

Coach's Tip: Supplements can fill small gaps, but they

Hydration: The Forgotten Nutrient

Dehydration sabotages progress more than most people realize.

If you don't drink enough water, you may experience:

- Lower strength and endurance

- Slower metabolism

- Increased cravings and fatigue

💡 Aim for about **half your bodyweight in ounces per day.** Example: 180 lbs → ~90 oz water daily (more if you sweat heavily).

Micronutrients

NUTRIENT	FUNCTIONS	FOOD SOURCES
Vitamin A	Vision, immune function	Carrots, sweet potatoes, spinach
Vitamin C	Immune function antioxidant	Citrus fruits, strawberries, bell peppers
Vitamin D	Bone health	Sunlight, fortified foods, fatty fish
Vitamin E	Antioxidant	Nuts, seeds, vegetable oils
Vitamin K	Blood clotting	Leafy greens, broccoli
Calcium	Bone health	Dairy products, fortified plant milks
Iron	Red blood cell formation	Red meat, beans, fortified cereals
Magnesium	Energy production, muscle function	Nuts, seeds, whole grains
Zinc	Immune function, wound healing	Meat, shelifish, legumes
Iodine	Thyroid function	Iodized salt, seafood

Micronutrients: The Silent Heroes

Macros (protein, carbs, fat) get all the attention, but **vitamins and minerals** are critical too.

- **Iron:** Transports oxygen to muscles (low iron = fatigue).

- **Magnesium:** Supports muscle recovery and sleep.

- **Vitamin D:** Helps bones, immunity, mood.

- **Fiber:** Regulates digestion and hunger.

☞ Best approach: eat a rainbow of fruits and veggies daily. Color = nutrients.

Timing: When to Eat for Performance

You don't need to obsess over six meals a day or "no food after 8pm." Total intake matters more than timing.

Still, some strategies help:

- **Pre-workout snack:** Light carbs + some protein (banana + yogurt, oats + protein powder).

- **Post-workout meal:** Protein + carbs to jumpstart recovery (chicken + rice, protein shake + fruit, eggs + toast).

Practical Eating Framework

Forget complicated calorie tracking (unless you enjoy it). Use the **Plate Method**:

- ½ plate = veggies and fruit

- ¼ plate = lean protein

- ¼ plate = whole carbs

- Add healthy fats (olive oil, nuts, avocado)

☞ This keeps meals balanced without obsessing over numbers.

🎁 Sidebar: Meal Prep Made Simple

1. **Cook protein in bulk.** (Chicken, lentils, or tofu for the week)

2. **Pre-chop veggies.** Store in containers for quick meals.

3. **Double dinner.** Tonight's meal = tomorrow's lunch.

4. **Snack smart.** Keep almonds, fruit, or Greek yogurt ready to grab.

Consistency comes from planning ahead—not winging it.

Coach's Note

When I finally stopped chasing fad diets and started

focusing on **protein, balance, and consistency**, everything changed.

I realized I wasn't "bad at dieting"—I was just under-eating protein and over-eating empty calories. Fixing that balance made results almost automatic.

Hydration was another game-changer. The day I started hitting my water goals, I felt stronger, had fewer cravings, and recovered faster.

☞ My best advice: don't aim for perfection. Track your food for one week—not to restrict yourself, but to **learn where your calories and protein actually land.** Most people are shocked at how little protein they eat compared to how many snack calories sneak in. Awareness is the first step to progress.

Inspirational Quote

"Take care of your body. It's the only place you have to live." – Jim Rohn

Chapter 6 – 30-Minute Dumbbell Workout

If I could only choose one piece of equipment for fat loss, strength, and versatility, it would be **dumbbells**. They're simple, effective, and adaptable for every fitness level. With just one pair and 30 minutes, you can work every major muscle group, torch calories, and walk away feeling accomplished.

This workout is designed to hit your **legs, chest, back, shoulders, arms, and core** while keeping your heart rate elevated. That means you're not just building muscle — you're also creating an afterburn effect (EPOC), where your metabolism stays revved up for hours after you finish.

Warm-Up (3 minutes)

A good warm-up primes your joints, raises your heart rate, and lowers injury risk.

- Arm circles – 30 seconds forward, 30 seconds backward

- Bodyweight squats – 10 reps

- Push-ups (knee or full) – 5 reps

- March in place with high knees – 1 minute

☞ Think of this as "switching on" your body. Warm muscles contract more efficiently and recover faster.

The Workout: Full-Body Dumbbell Circuit

Perform the following moves **circuit style**: complete one set of each exercise back-to-back with minimal rest. After finishing all six, rest 2 minutes. Repeat for **3 total rounds**.

1. Dumbbell Squat to Press (Thrusters)

- **Muscles worked:** Legs, shoulders, core

- **How to:** Hold dumbbells at shoulder height. Squat down with chest tall, then drive upward, pressing weights overhead in one motion.

- **Reps:** 10–12

- **Common mistakes:** Knees caving in, heels lifting, arching the lower back during press.

- **Progressions:** Use heavier weights, pause at bottom of squat.

- **Regressions:** Perform bodyweight squat → separate dumbbell press.

2. Dumbbell Bent-Over Rows

- **Muscles worked:** Back, biceps

- **How to:** Hinge at hips, keep back flat, dumbbells hanging near knees. Pull weights toward waist, squeeze shoulder blades.

- **Reps:** 10–12

- **Common mistakes:** Rounding spine, pulling only with arms.

- **Progressions:** Use heavier dumbbells or single-arm rows.

- **Regressions:** Support one hand on a bench/chair for stability.

3. Dumbbell Bench Press (or Floor Press)

- **Muscles worked:** Chest, shoulders, triceps

- **How to:** Lie flat on bench or floor. Press dumbbells straight up, then lower slowly until elbows bend to 90°.

- **Reps:** 10–12

- **Common mistakes:** Flaring elbows too wide, bouncing weights.

- **Progressions:** Add a slow 3–4 second lowering phase.

- **Regressions:** Press one dumbbell at a time with lighter weight.

4. Dumbbell Deadlifts

- **Muscles worked:** Hamstrings, glutes, lower back

- **How to:** Stand tall, dumbbells in front of thighs. Hinge at hips with flat back until weights reach shins. Drive up by squeezing glutes.

- **Reps:** 10–12

- **Common mistakes:** Turning it into a squat (knees too bent) or rounding spine.

- **Progressions:** Romanian deadlifts (slower, deeper stretch).

- **Regressions:** Use one dumbbell vertically, both hands gripping.

5. Dumbbell Shoulder Press

- **Muscles worked:** Shoulders, triceps

- **How to:** Sit or stand tall, press dumbbells overhead with palms forward. Keep core braced—no back arching.

- **Reps:** 10–12

- **Common mistakes:** Leaning back, shrugging shoulders.

- **Progressions:** Arnold press (rotate palms during press).

- **Regressions:** Alternate pressing one dumbbell at a time.

6. Dumbbell Bicep Curls

- **Muscles worked:** Biceps

- **How to:** Keep elbows close, curl weights slowly, lower with control.

- **Reps:** 12–15

- **Common mistakes:** Swinging or using momentum.

- **Progressions:** Hammer curls or slow tempo curls.

- **Regressions:** Lighter dumbbells, one arm at a time.

Dumbbell Workout Chart

Exercise	Sets	Reps	Notes
Squat to Press	3	10–12	Full-body power move
Dumbbell Bench/Floor Press	3	10–12	Lower slowly, avoid bounce
Bent-Over Rows	3	10–12	Keep back flat, squeeze lats
Dumbbell Deadlifts	3	10–12	Hinge hips, don't round spine
Shoulder Press	3	10–12	Core tight, don't arch back
Bicep Curls	2–3	12–15	Controlled tempo, no swinging
Plank (optional)	3	30 sec	Keep hips steady, core braced

FULL-BODY DUMBBELL CIRCUIT

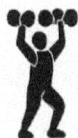

SQUAT TO PRESS
LEGS, SHOULDERS

DEADLIFT
LEGS, GLUTES

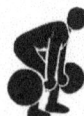

BENT-OVER ROW
BACK, BICEPS

CHEST PRESS
CHEST, TRICEPS

BICEP CURL
BICEPS

PLANK
CORE

Cool Down (3 minutes)

- Standing hamstring stretch – 30 sec per side

- Shoulder stretch across chest – 30 sec per side

- Overhead triceps stretch – 30 sec per side

- Deep breathing – 1 minute

☞ Cooling down improves flexibility and signals your body it's safe to recover.

Why This Works

This circuit blends **compound lifts** (squats, rows, deadlifts, presses) with isolation (biceps, shoulders) to hit every muscle. The compound moves torch calories and build functional strength; the isolation moves shape and balance your physique.

Because it's structured as a circuit, your **heart rate stays high**, meaning you're getting cardio benefits while lifting. Add progressive overload—slightly more weight, reps, or slower tempo—and you'll unlock steady fat loss and lean muscle growth.

Coach's Note

When I first started lifting with dumbbells, I made the mistake of chasing heavy weights too soon. My form suffered, and instead of progress, I got stuck. Once I slowed down, focused on **form first, weight second**, and added intensity gradually, my results exploded.

☞ Remember: you don't need fancy variations. Master these six moves. If you can squat, row, press, curl, and deadlift well, you'll build a strong, athletic, lean body faster than if you scattered your energy across 50 random exercises.

Progression doesn't only mean adding weight. Try slowing the tempo, pausing at the hardest point, or cutting rest times. Consistency + control will always beat recklessness.

Inspirational Quote

"The day you think there is no improvement to be made, is a sad one for any player." – Lionel Messi

Chapter 7 – 30-Minute Resistance Band Workout

Resistance bands are one of the most **underrated tools in fitness**. They're portable, affordable, joint-friendly, and deceptively effective. Whether you're traveling, working out at home, or just craving variety, bands can give you a **full-body, calorie-torching session** in just 30 minutes.

I used to dismiss bands as "beginner gear" or just for rehab. But once I trained seriously with them, I realized how effective they are. Bands keep muscles under **constant tension**, unlike dumbbells that allow "rest" at the top of a move. This extra stress builds strength, endurance, and tone faster than you might expect.

Warm-Up (3 minutes)

This quick sequence wakes up your joints and preps the muscles you'll train:

- Band pull-aparts – 10 reps (great for posture and shoulder stability)

- Bodyweight squats – 10 reps (to activate glutes and quads)

- Arm swings forward & backward – 30 seconds each

- March in place with high knees – 1 minute

☞ Bands aren't just workout tools—they also supercharge your warm-up by improving mobility and activating stabilizer muscles.

The Workout: Full-Body Resistance Band Circuit

Like the dumbbell workout, this is a **circuit**. Perform one set of each move back-to-back. Rest 2 minutes after completing all six. Repeat for **3 rounds total**.

1. Band Squats

- **Muscles worked:** Legs, glutes

- **How to:** Stand on the band, hold handles at shoulders. Sit back into a squat, then drive upward through your heels.

- **Reps:** 12–15

- **Common mistakes:** Knees collapsing inward, rounding lower back.

- **Progressions:** Use a thicker band, pause at the bottom.

- **Regressions:** Do bodyweight squats or place band above knees for lighter tension.

2. Band Chest Press

- **Muscles worked:** Chest, shoulders, triceps

- **How to:** Anchor the band behind you at chest height. Step forward for tension, press handles straight ahead, return with control.

- **Reps:** 10–12

- **Common mistakes:** Shrugging shoulders, letting the band snap back.

- **Progressions:** Heavier band, or single-arm presses.

- **Regressions:** Step closer to anchor for lighter resistance.

3. Band Rows

- **Muscles worked:** Back, biceps

- **How to:** Anchor band at waist height. Pull handles toward your torso, squeeze shoulder blades together.

- **Reps:** 10–12

- **Common mistakes:** Hunching shoulders, pulling with arms only.

- **Progressions:** Heavier band, slower 3-second squeeze.

- **Regressions:** Anchor under feet and row seated.

4. Band Overhead Press

- **Muscles worked:** Shoulders, triceps

- **How to:** Stand on band, handles at shoulders. Press overhead without arching back.

- **Reps:** 10–12

- **Common mistakes:** Overarching spine, flaring ribs.

- **Progressions:** Heavier band or add pulses at top.

- **Regressions:** Press one arm at a time or use lighter band.

5. Band Pull-Aparts

- **Muscles worked:** Upper back, rear shoulders

- **How to:** Hold band at chest height, arms straight. Pull apart until arms are wide, return slowly.

- **Reps:** 12–15

- **Common mistakes:** Bending elbows, shrugging shoulders.

- **Progressions:** Shorten grip (choke up) or use stronger band.

- **Regressions:** Light band, higher reps (15–20).

6. Band Side Steps (Glute Burnout)

- **Muscles worked:** Glutes, hips

- **How to:** Place band above knees or ankles. Step side-to-side while keeping knees bent.

- **Reps:** 10–12 steps each way

- **Common mistakes:** Standing too tall, letting knees cave inward.

- **Progressions:** Heavier band, or hold squat position during steps.

- **Regressions:** Smaller steps, band above knees.

Band Workout Chart

Exercise	Sets	Reps/Steps	Notes
Band Squats	3	12–15	Stand on band, full squat
Band Chest Press	3	10–12	Anchor behind, press forward
Band Rows	3	10–12	Anchor waist height, squeeze lats
Band Overhead Press	3	10–12	Core tight, avoid arching back
Band Pull-Aparts	2–3	12–15	Arms straight, control movement
Band Side Steps	3	10–12 steps/side	Low squat, steady tension

CHAPTER 7 – 30-MINUTE RESISTANCE BAND WORKOUT CICUIT

BAND SQUATS
LEGS

BAND CHEST PRESS
CHEST

BAND ROWS
BACK

BAND OVERHEAD PRESS
SHOULDERS

BAND PULL-APARTS
SHOULDERS

BAND SIDE STEPS
GLUTES

Cool Down (3 minutes)

- Shoulder stretch across chest – 30 sec each side

- Chest opener (hands clasped behind back) – 30 sec

- Seated hamstring stretch – 30 sec each side

- Deep breathing – 1 minute

☞ Stretching with the same bands adds gentle resistance, helping muscles recover faster.

Why This Works

Resistance bands provide **variable resistance**—the further you stretch, the harder it gets. This keeps muscles under tension through the **entire range of motion**, something dumbbells can't always do.

Bands also protect your joints by eliminating heavy compressive forces. They're perfect for building strength, endurance, and tone without pounding your body. Plus, because they're portable, you can train **anywhere, anytime**.

Coach's Note

I used to see bands as "too easy." Then I tried a band circuit on the road and realized how wrong I was. My muscles were burning, my form had to be strict, and the pump was incredible. Bands taught me that tension—not weight—drives results.

☞ If you want to grow stronger, don't just go heavier. Go slower. Pause under tension. Focus on the squeeze. With bands, those small tweaks make a massive difference.

Inspirational Quote

"No matter how good you get, you can always get better, and that's the exciting part." – Tiger Woods

Chapter 8 – 30-Minute Bodyweight Workout

Here's the truth: you don't need fancy equipment to get in shape. **Your body is the best piece of equipment you'll ever own.** With bodyweight training, you can build muscle, burn fat, and improve endurance anywhere—your living room, a hotel, or outdoors at the park.

I love bodyweight workouts because they remove excuses. No dumbbells? No bands? No problem. If you've got **30 minutes and some open space**, you can get a challenging workout that improves strength, stability, and conditioning.

Why Bodyweight Training Works

Even without external weights, bodyweight training is brutally effective. Here's why:

1. **Progressive Overload Still Applies** – You can increase difficulty by slowing tempo, adding reps, shortening rest, or moving to harder variations (push-ups → diamond push-ups → plyometric push-ups).

2. **Core & Stability Engagement** – Controlling your body through space forces stabilizer muscles to activate, building balance and athleticism.

3. **Strength + Cardio in One** – Circuit-style training elevates heart rate like HIIT while still building lean muscle, delivering a double benefit.

Warm-Up (3 minutes)

A quick prep routine to activate muscles and increase blood flow:

- Jumping jacks – 1 minute

- High knees – 30 seconds

- Arm circles – 30 seconds each way

- Air squats – 10 reps

☞ Warm-ups matter: they increase performance and lower injury risk.

The Workout: Full-Body Bodyweight Circuit

Perform each move back-to-back with minimal rest. After all 6 exercises, rest for **90 seconds**. Complete **3 rounds total.**

1. Push-Ups

- **Muscles worked:** Chest, shoulders, triceps, core

- **How to:** Hands under shoulders, body in straight line. Lower until chest nearly touches floor, then press up.

- **Reps:** 8–12

- **Common mistakes:** Sagging hips, flaring elbows.

- **Progressions:** Decline push-ups, clap push-ups.

- **Regressions:** Knee push-ups, wall push-ups.

2. Squats

- **Muscles worked:** Legs, glutes

- **How to:** Feet shoulder-width apart. Sit back like into a chair, chest tall, push through heels.

- **Reps:** 12–15

- **Common mistakes:** Knees caving in, heels lifting.

- **Progressions:** Jump squats, pistol squats.

- **Regressions:** Half squats, sit-to-chair squats.

3. Lunges

- **Muscles worked:** Quads, hamstrings, glutes, core

- **How to:** Step forward, lower until both knees at 90°, push back to start. Alternate legs.

- **Reps:** 10 per leg

- **Common mistakes:** Leaning torso forward, stepping too far.

- **Progressions:** Jumping lunges.

- **Regressions:** Static lunges (stay in place).

4. Glute Bridges

- **Muscles worked:** Glutes, hamstrings, lower back

- **How to:** Lie on back, knees bent. Drive through heels to lift hips, squeeze glutes at the top.

- **Reps:** 12–15

- **Common mistakes:** Overarching lower back.

- **Progressions:** Single-leg glute bridges.

- **Regressions:** Partial bridges, short range of motion.

5. Sit-Ups / Crunches

- **Muscles worked:** Core, hip flexors

- **How to:** Lie on back, knees bent. Curl torso up toward thighs, lower with control.

- **Reps:** 12–15

- **Common mistakes:** Pulling on neck, using momentum.

- **Progressions:** V-ups, bicycles.

- **Regressions:** Small crunches, hands across chest.

6. Plank Shoulder Taps

- **Muscles worked:** Core, shoulders

- **How to:** Hold plank, tap right hand to left shoulder, then left to right. Keep hips steady.

- **Reps:** 10 per side

- **Common mistakes:** Rocking hips side to side.

- **Progressions:** Extended-arm plank, arm reach.

- **Regressions:** Standard plank hold.

Body Workout Chart

Exercise	Sets	Reps/Time	Notes
Push-Ups	3	8–12	Modify on knees if needed
Squats	3	12–15	Push through heels, chest tall
Lunges	3	10/leg	Knees at 90°, don't lean fwd
Glute Bridges	3	12–15	Squeeze glutes at top
Sit-Ups / Crunches	3	12–15	Controlled, no pulling neck
Plank Shoulder Taps	3	10/side	Keep hips steady

30-MINUTE BODYWEIGHT WORKOUT

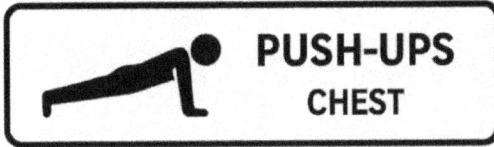

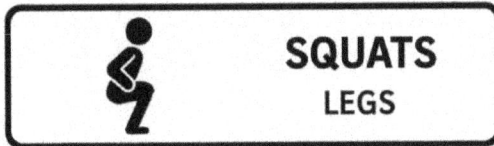

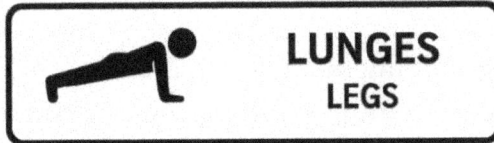

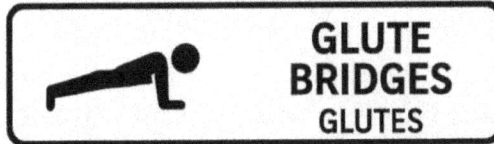

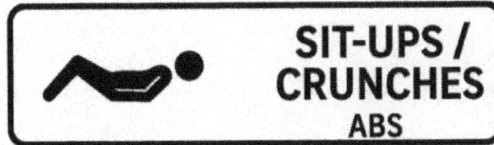

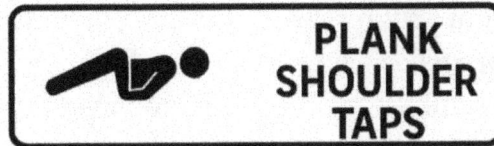

PUSH-UPS
CHEST

SQUATS
LEGS

LUNGES
LEGS

GLUTE BRIDGES
GLUTES

SIT-UPS / CRUNCHES
ABS

PLANK SHOULDER TAPS

Cool Down (3 minutes)

- Quad stretch – 30 sec each side

- Hamstring stretch – 30 sec each side

- Shoulder stretch – 30 sec each side

- Deep breathing – 1 minute

☞ Cooling down improves recovery and flexibility, preparing you for your next session.

Why This Works

Bodyweight training builds more than strength—it develops **coordination, stability, and endurance**. Circuits elevate heart rate like cardio, but the focus on controlled movement still tones and strengthens muscles.

It's scalable, meaning you can **start as a beginner** and progress toward advanced moves, all without needing any equipment.

Coach's Note

There were times when I didn't have access to a gym. At first, I thought progress would stop—but bodyweight workouts proved me wrong. Done with intensity and good form, they humbled me and delivered results.

☞ Don't underestimate these moves. Control the tempo,

use a full range of motion, and push yourself. Even today, when life gets busy, I return to bodyweight basics. They remind me: fitness isn't about equipment—it's about effort and consistency.

Inspirational Quote

"Don't count the days, make the days count." – Muhammad Ali

Chapter 9 – Mixing It Up: How to Choose the Right Workout for You

Why Variety Matters

If there's one truth I've learned in 20+ years of training, it's this: boredom kills consistency. Doing the same workout on repeat may feel safe and familiar, but over time it dulls both your motivation and your results.

Here's why:

- **Adaptation Principle** – Your body becomes efficient at repeated tasks. The same workout that once felt challenging now burns fewer calories and stimulates less muscle growth.

- **Plateaus Happen** – When your body adapts, progress slows or stalls. Without new challenges, you risk frustration and burnout.

- **The Engagement Factor** – Fresh workouts keep your mind and body stimulated, which makes it far easier to stay consistent long term.

☞ Think of variety not as "confusing your muscles," but as

reminding them they have more to give.

The Science of Adaptation and Progression

Your muscles and nervous system thrive on challenge. The trick is balancing **consistency** (sticking with resistance training) with **variety** (rotating exercises, tools, and intensity).

- **Progressive Overload** → Increasing weight, reps, sets, or intensity over time keeps muscles growing.

- **Periodization** → Planned variation in your training (weekly, monthly, or seasonally) prevents overuse and ensures long-term progress.

- **Neuromuscular Adaptation** → Trying new tools like bands or bodyweight drills recruits stabilizer muscles that dumbbells might miss.

Think of it like shifting gears in a car. Staying in first gear forever won't take you far. Switching gears strategically allows you to accelerate smoothly and keep moving forward.

Choosing the Right Workout for Your Day

You don't need a complex plan—you just need to know which tool fits best into your circumstances. Here's a quick guide:

- **If you're at home with dumbbells or at the gym →** Do the **Dumbbell Workout (Ch. 6).**

- **If you're traveling or want joint-friendly variety →** Do the **Resistance Band Workout (Ch. 7).**

- **If you have zero equipment or limited space →** Do the **Bodyweight Workout (Ch. 8).**

Sample Weekly Rotations

Here are some proven structures depending on your fitness level and schedule:

2-Day Routine (Beginner)

- Day 1: Dumbbell Workout

- Day 2: Bodyweight Workout
  ☞ Plus walking on in-between days.

3-Day Routine (Intermediate)

- Monday: Dumbbell Workout

- Wednesday: Bodyweight Workout

- Friday: Resistance Band Workout

4-Day Routine (Advanced)

- Monday: Dumbbell Workout

- Tuesday: Bodyweight Workout

- Thursday: Resistance Band Workout

- Saturday: Dumbbell Workout (repeat for strength emphasis)

☞ The exact days matter less than the balance. Rotate tools and give yourself rest.

Why Walking Fits Into Every Plan

Walking is the ultimate recovery tool between resistance workouts. Unlike high-intensity cardio, it:

- Burns fat as a primary fuel source at lower intensities.

- Lowers cortisol (your stress hormone), which helps reduce belly fat.

- Boosts circulation, aiding muscle recovery.

- Supports consistency—you can walk daily without strain.

💡 *Pro tip: Outdoor walking multiplies benefits with sunlight (vitamin D), mood boosts, and mental clarity.*

📖 **Sidebar: The Power of Outdoor Walking**

◎ **Stress Reduction** – Nature walks lower cortisol more effectively than indoor activity.

☀◎ **Vitamin D Boost** – Sunlight supports bones, immunity, and mood.

◎ **Mental Clarity** – Green spaces improve focus,

creativity, and mental health.

♥◉ **Faster Recovery** – Gentle outdoor walking promotes blood flow and healing.

☞ Bottom line: A 30-minute outdoor walk is more than calorie burn—it's therapy for body and mind.

Mini Challenges to Break Plateaus

Short challenges inject fun and help you break out of ruts. Try one when motivation dips:

- **Push-Up Power Week** → Add 10 push-ups at the end of every workout.

- **Step Count Challenge** → Add 2,000 steps to your daily average for one week.

- **Tempo Training Week** → Slow every rep (3 seconds down, 1 pause, explosive up).

- **Core Every Day Week** → Add one short ab exercise daily.

☞ Small, structured experiments create excitement without derailing your overall program.

Coach's Note

When I replaced "mandatory runs" with variety—mixing dumbbells, bands, bodyweight, and outdoor walks—everything changed. My body responded faster, my joints felt better, and I actually *looked forward* to training again.

The secret isn't chasing the newest fad—it's balancing consistency with enough variation to stay challenged. When you feel stuck, don't quit. Switch things up. That's how you'll keep progressing for years to come.

Inspirational Quote

"The body achieves what the mind believes." – Unknown

Chapter 10 – Staying Motivated and Consistent

Motivation is a funny thing. Some days you wake up ready to crush your workout, and other days just getting off the couch feels impossible. Here's the truth: you won't always feel motivated. But that's not a problem—because motivation isn't what transforms your body. **Habits and consistency are.**

Think of motivation as the spark that lights the fire, but habits as the wood that keeps it burning. When habits are in place, you don't need to rely on feelings—you just follow the system you've built.

Why Motivation Fades

Motivation is tied to emotion. It spikes when you're excited about something new—a fresh goal, a new gym membership, a challenge with friends—but it dips as soon as the novelty wears off. Psychologists call this the **motivation curve**, and you've probably seen it in action:

- Gyms are packed in January when everyone is excited about resolutions.

- By March, the crowd thins out.

That's because excitement wears off. What keeps people going long-term isn't motivation—it's **systems, routines, and identity-based habits.**

The Habit Loop: Cue → Routine → Reward

Building consistency means working with your brain's wiring. Every habit follows a simple loop:

1. **Cue** – A trigger that reminds you to act. (Example: laying out workout clothes the night before.)

2. **Routine** – The action itself. (Your 30-minute workout.)

3. **Reward** – The benefit your brain craves. (The endorphins, energy boost, or simply the pride of finishing.)

Over time, your brain starts craving the reward, which makes the routine feel automatic. That's why the hardest part is starting—the habit loop gets easier the longer you stick with it.

Practical Ways to Stay Consistent (When Motivation Fails)

1. **Treat Workouts Like Appointments**

Block time in your calendar. If it's scheduled, it's harder to skip. Think of it like a meeting with your future self.

2. **Start Smaller Than You Think**
   If you're struggling, commit to just 10 minutes. Most of the time, once you start, momentum carries you through the full session.

3. **Track Progress Beyond the Scale**
   Use a notebook, app, or simple calendar. Check off workouts, track strength gains, or take monthly progress photos. Seeing results fuels consistency.

4. **Leverage Accountability**
   Tell a friend, post online, or join a class. Humans stick to commitments better when someone else is involved.

5. **Stack Habits**
   Attach a new habit to an existing one. Example: after morning coffee, do 20 squats. The brain loves linking routines.

6. **Shape Your Environment**
   Make good habits easy and bad habits harder. Keep dumbbells in your living room, place a yoga mat by your bed, or prep workout clothes before bed.

7. **Celebrate Every Win**
   Finishing a workout—even a short one—is a victory. Reward yourself with something positive (a walk outdoors, new gear, or even just a moment to reflect).

The Psychology of Missing Workouts

Here's something critical: **missing one workout isn't failure—it's feedback.** The real danger is letting one missed day snowball into a week, then a month.

Instead of guilt, use curiosity: *Why did I skip? Was it time, energy, stress?* Learn from it and adjust. If you miss, don't double up or punish yourself—just return the next day.

☞ **Consistency is not about perfection. It's about always coming back.**

Mindset Shifts That Build Resilience

- **From Chore → Gift**: Workouts aren't punishment—they're an investment in your future self.

- **From All-or-Nothing → Progress**: Two workouts a week beat zero. Consistency stacks up.

- **From Short-Term → Lifestyle**: Fitness isn't a 6-week challenge. It's a lifetime practice.

Once you shift your identity from "someone trying to lose weight" to "someone who trains," the rest follows naturally.

Coach's Note

I've been training for over 20 years, and I still have days where I don't feel like it. The difference now is that I don't wait for motivation—I rely on habits. I treat my workouts like brushing my teeth. It's not optional; it's just part of my day.

There was a season when life was overwhelming—work deadlines, family obligations, stress piling up. I missed nearly two weeks of training. Old me would have quit. New me leaned on the **habit loop**. I told myself: *"Just put on your shoes and start."* That tiny step was the cue. Once I started, the rest followed, and the reward was feeling alive again.

My personal fallback routine is simple: when I need to reestablish consistency, I go back to the **full-body dumbbell workout** from Chapter 6. Three or four days a week of that circuit, paired with daily walking, always resets me. It reminds me that fitness isn't about perfection—it's about rhythm.

☞ Feel free to experiment and find what works for you. The best plan is the one you'll actually stick to.

🎁 Sidebar: 30-Day Consistency Challenge

Want to lock in the habit of training? Try this structured challenge.

Your Mission

- Complete **12 resistance workouts** (Chapters 6–8) in 30 days.

- Walk **every day** for 20–30 minutes.

Weekly Focus

- **Week 1** → Just show up.

- **Week 2** → Add intensity (extra reps, more weight, or shorter rest).

- **Week 3** → Make it automatic. Training feels like part of your day.

- **Week 4** → Reflect and reset. Celebrate, then roll momentum into the next month.

☞ **Coach's Tip:** Don't focus on "never missing." Focus on "never quitting." Even 70% completion beats 0%.

Inspirational Quote

"Discipline is doing what you hate to do, but nonetheless doing it like you love it." – Mike Tyson

Conclusion – Stronger Every Day

You've made it to the end of this journey—but in many ways, this is just the beginning. The real value of what you've learned isn't in reading these chapters; it's in applying them. Every rep, every step, every meal, and every choice adds up to something greater: a stronger, healthier, more confident you.

What You've Learned

Over these chapters, you've built a toolkit for lifelong fitness:

- **Why Resistance Training Wins** → Builds muscle, burns fat after you finish, and reshapes your body like cardio never can.

- **The Role of Nutrition** → Calories and protein drive results, but balance and sustainability keep them alive.

- **The Power of Recovery** → Sleep, walking, and active rest are as vital as lifting weights.

- **Consistency & Habits** → Systems, not motivation,

are the foundation of long-term success.

Think of it as a four-legged table: **Training, Nutrition, Recovery, and Consistency.** If even one is missing, the table wobbles. When all four are strong, your foundation is unshakable.

Beyond the Scale

It's easy to obsess over numbers—weight, calories, reps, or even the scale itself. But your true progress shows up in how you feel and live:

- Your clothes fitting more comfortably.

- The confidence you carry into work, family, and relationships.

- The strength you feel in daily life—lifting groceries, climbing stairs, or simply standing taller.

- The energy that spills over into everything you do.

💡 **Mindset Shift:** Stop chasing a number. Start chasing strength, confidence, and consistency.

Identity Shift – Becoming the Athlete of Your Own Life

This book isn't just about workouts; it's about identity. You're no longer "someone trying to lose weight." You're someone who trains. Someone who takes ownership of their health. Someone who builds strength in the gym, in the kitchen, and in life.

When you shift your identity, the habits follow naturally. Athletes train. Athletes fuel their bodies. Athletes rest with purpose. And now—you are that athlete.

Your Next Steps

Don't close this book and wait for the "perfect" time to start. The best time is now.
Here's your action plan:

1. **Pick Your Workout Schedule** → 2, 3, or 4 days a week (see Appendix).

2. **Walk Daily** → Even 20 minutes counts. Outdoors if possible.

3. **Fuel Smart** → Prioritize protein, balance carbs and fats, hydrate.

4. **Rest Intentionally** → 7–8 hours of sleep, plus active recovery.

5. **Track Progress** → Strength gains, photos, and how you *feel* matter more than the scale.

📖 Sidebar: Core Lessons Recap

- Resistance training = best tool for fat loss & body recomposition.

- Protein = the foundation of nutrition.

- Walking = recovery + fat burning without stress.

- Sleep = the ultimate "secret weapon."

- Consistency beats perfection. Always.

Coach's Final Note

I've been where you are—frustrated, stuck, and chasing the wrong things. I tried the fad diets, the endless cardio, and the shortcuts. None of it worked long-term. What did work was simple: **lift, fuel, walk, rest, repeat.**

There's no magic pill. There's only the choice to keep showing up. Some days you'll crush it. Some days you'll barely get through. Both count. Both move you forward.

☞ My advice: Don't quit. Ever. If you fall off for a week, a month, or even a year—just get back up. Fitness isn't about being perfect. It's about coming back, over and over, until showing up is simply who you are.

This is more than fitness. It's freedom. And it's yours.

Inspirational Quote

"Champions keep playing until they get it right." – *Billie Jean King*

Appendix – Your Quick-Start Handbook

The main chapters of this book give you the *why* and the *how*. The Appendix is here to give you the *what*—practical plans, charts, and guides you can use immediately. Think of it as your reference toolkit: everything you need to get started without second-guessing yourself.

Quick Start Workout Plans

Sometimes the hardest part is knowing where to begin. These plans remove the guesswork by showing you how to plug the Dumbbell (Ch. 6), Resistance Band (Ch. 7), and Bodyweight (Ch. 8) workouts into your week.

2-Day Plan (Beginner Friendly)

This is the "minimum effective dose." Great if you're new or have a tight schedule.

- **Day 1:** Dumbbell Workout

- **Day 2:** Walk (20–40 min at easy pace)

- **Day 3:** Bodyweight Workout

- **Day 4:** Walk outdoors (20–40 min)

- **Day 5:** Rest

- **Day 6:** Walk

- **Day 7:** Rest

☞ Why it works: Even 2 resistance workouts per week build muscle, while walking fills in recovery and fat burning.

Progression Ideas:

- Add a 4th round to your circuits.

- Slowly increase dumbbell weight every 2–3 weeks.

- Add a mini-challenge: e.g., 30-sec plank or 10 extra push-ups.

3-Day Plan (Intermediate)

This is the sweet spot for most people—enough training to see rapid results without burnout.

- **Day 1:** Dumbbell Workout

- **Day 2:** Walk (20–45 min)

- **Day 3:** Bodyweight Workout

- **Day 4:** Rest or walk

- **Day 5:** Resistance Band Workout

- **Day 6:** Walk outdoors (30–60 min)

- **Day 7:** Rest

☞ Why it works: 3 lifting sessions per week keeps your muscles stimulated, while walks aid recovery and fat burning.

Progression Ideas:

- Add supersets (two moves back-to-back).

- Slow down tempo (3–4 sec lowering).

- Try harder variations (e.g., push-ups → decline push-ups).

4-Day Plan (Advanced)

For those ready to commit more intensity and volume.

- **Day 1:** Dumbbell Workout

- **Day 2:** Walk (20–40 min)

- **Day 3:** Resistance Band Workout

- **Day 4:** Long Walk outdoors (45–60 min)

- **Day 5:** Dumbbell Workout (repeat, heavier focus)

- **Day 6:** Bodyweight Workout

- **Day 7:** Rest

☞ Why it works: 4 lifting days accelerate fat loss, strength, and conditioning while keeping recovery intact.

Progression Ideas:

- Occasionally add a 5th workout if fully recovered.

- Increase resistance with heavier dumbbells or thicker bands.

- Insert a mini-challenge week (push-up week, step count goal, tempo week).

Macronutrients and Their Energy Value

Every calorie you eat comes from one of three macronutrients: protein, carbonydrates, and fats. Each has a different energy value and effect on your metabolism.

Macronutrient	Calories per Gram	Thermic Effect of Food	Key Role in Fitness
Protein	4 kcal/g	~20-30%	Muscle repair
Carbs	4 kcal/g	~5-10%	satiety metab- bism
Fat	9 kcal/g	0-3%	energy reserve

☞ Notice that protein not only supports muscle, but also takes the most energy to digest. That means eating higher-protein meals actually helps you burn more calories throughout the day.

Nutrition Reference Charts

Nutrition is the other half of the puzzle. This section

simplifies daily needs into clear charts.

Calorie & Protein Guidelines

- **Men (18–30 yrs):** ~2,600–2,800 kcal (maintenance); 2,100–2,300 for fat loss.

- **Women (18–30 yrs):** ~2,000–2,200 kcal (maintenance); 1,500–1,700 for fat loss.

- **Protein:** 0.7–1.0 g per lb bodyweight.

☞ Example: A 180 lb person should aim for 125–180 g protein daily.

Flexible Options & Tips

- **Vegetarian swaps:** Chickpeas, lentils, tofu, seitan, edamame in place of meat.

- **Snack swaps:**

  ○ Sweet craving → protein smoothie, fruit with yogurt.

  ○ Savory craving → hummus with veggies, roasted chickpeas.

- **Meal prep hacks:**

  ○ Cook proteins in bulk (chicken, beef, lentils).

  ○ Prep veggies ahead for grab-and-go meals.

  ○ Double dinner portions → next day's lunch.

Grocery List (Quick Reference)

Proteins: Chicken, turkey, lean beef, eggs, Greek yogurt,
cottage cheese, salmon, tuna, beans, tofu.
Carbs: Brown rice, oats, quinoa, whole wheat bread/pasta,
sweet potatoes, fruit.
Fats: Olive oil, avocado, nuts, seeds, peanut butter, fish oil.
Veggies: Broccoli, spinach, asparagus, carrots, cucumbers,
peppers, mixed greens.

Hydration Guidelines

- **Baseline:** Half your bodyweight in ounces daily
  (180 lbs = ~90 oz).

- **During intense training:** Add 12–16 oz per 30 min
  of heavy sweating.

- **Tip:** If you feel sluggish, crave sugar, or get
  headaches, dehydration may be the culprit.

Supplements Simplified

Supplements aren't required, but they can help.

Essential (if diet is lacking):

- **Whey Protein:** Convenient protein boost.

- **Creatine Monohydrate:** Increases strength and
  recovery.

- **Fish Oil (Omega-3):** Supports joints, heart, and brain.

- **Multivitamin:** Covers potential gaps.

Optional (nice-to-have):

- **Caffeine (coffee/pre-workout):** Boosts energy and focus.

- **Electrolytes:** Useful if training in hot climates or sweating heavily.

- **Greens Powder:** Fills in when fruit/veggie intake is low.

☞ Rule: Supplements should *supplement* a solid diet, not replace it.

7-Day Balanced Meal Plan (Sample)

A practical framework for a week. Portion sizes adjust to your needs.

- **Day 1:** Greek yogurt + berries; chicken + rice + broccoli; salmon + quinoa; almonds + apple.

- **Day 2:** Eggs + toast; turkey sandwich + carrots; beef stir-fry + rice; protein shake.

- **Day 3:** Oatmeal + banana; tuna salad; chicken fajitas; cottage cheese + walnuts.

- **Day 4:** Smoothie; quinoa salad + chickpeas; cod + sweet potato + asparagus; trail mix.

- **Day 5:** Boiled eggs + avocado toast; chicken wrap; turkey meatballs + pasta; protein bar.

- **Day 6:** Cottage cheese + strawberries; salmon bowl; roast chicken + sweet potatoes; apple + almonds.

- **Day 7:** Pancakes with fruit; grilled shrimp + quinoa; lean steak + baked potato + Brussels sprouts; yogurt parfait.

☞ Vegetarian swaps: tofu, lentils, beans, seitan for protein.

Practical Tools & Checklists

- **Plate Method (Meal Balance):** ½ veggies/fruit, ¼ protein, ¼ carbs + healthy fats.

- **Step Count Challenge:** Add +2,000 steps to your daily average for 4 weeks.

- **Mini Challenges (from Ch. 9):** Push-up week, tempo week, core challenge.

- **Tracking Progress:** Photos, strength log, step count—not just the scale.

🎁 Sidebar: The "Consistency Compass"
When in doubt, ask yourself:

1. Did I train (2–4x this week)?

2. Did I walk daily?

3. Did I prioritize protein?

4. Did I sleep 7–8 hrs?

If you hit at least 3 out of 4, you're on track.

Coach's Final Final Note

When I learned to treat food as fuel most of the time—and treats as just that, treats—it changed everything. I still enjoy pizza or dessert, but I plan them in, enjoy a portion, and move on. The key isn't perfection, it's **balance and consistency.**

And speaking of consistency, let me share what it looks like for me personally: when I'm on track, I almost always default to the **full-body dumbbell routine** (from Chapter 6). I'll run through it **3 to 4 days a week** because it's simple, efficient, and I know it hits all the major muscle groups. When I stay locked into that rhythm, paired with walking and balanced nutrition, I feel my best physically and mentally.

Feel free to experiment and find what works for you.

Final Inspirational Quotes

"Some people want it to happen, some wish it would happen, others make it happen." – *Michael Jordan*

🏆 "I've missed more than 9,000 shots in my career. I've lost almost 300 games. Twenty-six times I've been trusted to take the game-winning shot and missed. I've failed over and over and over again in my life. And that is why I succeed." – *Michael Jordan*

www.ingramcontent.com/pod-product-compliance
Lightning Source LLC
Chambersburg PA
CBHW032116280326
41933CB00009B/866